Heart
Nursing

Learn, Grow & Succeed
In The First Year of Practice

Amanda V. West

Heart Nursing:
Learn, Grow & Succeed
In The First Year of Practice

Copyright © 2012 by Amanda V. West

Smashwords Edition May 2012

Copyright © 2012 by Amanda V. West

All rights reserved.

ISBN: 1481178334
ISBN-13: 9781481178334

Library of Congress Control Number: XXXXX
LCCN Imprint Name: City and State

Contents

Acknowledgments

To the wonderful nurses who have been my teammates, teachers, leaders and friends...I say thank you. You've been shining examples to me of what the nursing profession is all about. I'm so grateful to be a part of it. To my family, thank you for your constant love and encouragement.

Lessons Learned

I recall my first year as a nurse. No book had taught me how to call doctors, how to hold ten thoughts in my head at any moment, or how to work a whole shift without going to the bathroom. On some days I thought, "How am I possibly going to finish all that I have to do? Am I really supposed to keep smiling when I'm this exhausted?" Most of all, I remember thinking that I must not have paid close attention in nursing school! Oh sure, everything made sense in the books, but putting it into practice was something else altogether.

Fast forward a few years into my pediatric nursing career. By then, I could organize my thoughts pretty well and complete multiple tasks in a timely fashion. I could even remember to pee during my shift! I must have picked up some decent nursing skills along the way, huh? Well, almost.

I learned the best lessons about being a great nurse when I practiced nursing from my heart. I will always remember the times when I cried with parents who received bad news about their child's health, jumped in to help my teammates when they needed me, or delayed my next task to play a game with my patients.

Over the course of the first year in practice as a nurse, you will have your share of classes, skill set checkoffs, orientations, and buddy shifts, designed to help you demonstrate competence and good old-fashioned know-how. To add to that, I hope to share with you some of the best lessons I learned as a student and as a new graduate, during on the job training. Some lessons are simple, of course, but they have set the stage for my nursing career and caused me to learn and grow as a nurse and a person. I'm sure they will do they will do the same for you.

1

Heart Nursing 101:
How Compassion Looks in Practice

Kindness is the language which the deaf can hear and the blind can see.

~Mark Twain

Sarah, a bright, young student, spends her Saturdays volunteering at a local nursing home. She enjoys spending time with the residents, listening to their stories and helping the nurses care for them. She one day decides, *I want to be a nurse.* With her love for comforting others, Sarah is on the road to becoming an incredible nurse to her patients. How do I know this? Keep reading!

Sarah is like so many of us when we decide to become nurses. I think we all at some point aspire to be "miracle workers". Perhaps the greatest ambition we have as nurses is to provide excellent care that, in turn, adds irreplaceable value to someone's life. Is it a high ambition? Sure and compassion is the key! What is tough at times is realizing the tremendous impact of compassion as a new nurse. When I started nursing practice, I thought I had done well by my patients when my medications were given on time! Compassion was not a new concept to me, but my view of nursing practice was completely revamped after I learned how it truly affected my care of patients. If your goal is to be a "miracle worker" to your patients, taking these lessons on compassion to heart is a great place to start.

First, compassion forms the nucleus of nursing care. It feeds into all of your tasks and goals as a nurse. Compassion is especially crucial in your shifts. You will work shifts that absolutely test the limits of your physical, mental, and emotional endurance. My colleagues and I call those shifts "trials by fire". During those times, your sympathy for your patients gives you the ability to push through. I remember caring for patients who kept me so busy that I missed lunch breaks! Yet, in the moments when I felt an emotional breakdown coming on, I thought of my patients' situations. That gave me the energy to go get more juice, bring more pain medication, or call the doctor again. I could keep going because I brought concern for my patients to the forefront of my mind.

Calling the doctor was the most nerve-racking part of my early nursing career. I would think, *What if I sound dumb?* or *I've spoken to him three times already.* You will experience this, too. Imagine that doctors' rounds are done. The doctor comes in to talk with the patient (or parents, if the patient is a child). Everyone's on the same page about the plan of care. You feel a good shift coming on. The doctor leaves and then the parents express concern that their child is still in pain and needs a different pain medication. Do you try to reassure the parents or do you bring their concerns to the doctor's attention? Let compassion decide for you. I guarantee that, if make compassion the center of your decision, you'll be astounded by the results. Courage wells up, especially when it's time to phone the doctor! Here's the bottom line. Sometimes the simple act of showing genuine concern can be much more helpful than all the medical knowledge in the world.

Compassion will also lay groundwork for the type of nurse you will be throughout your career. The field of nursing offers many career avenues. Whether you work as a case manager, forensic nurse, or nurse teacher, you'll have many chances to sympathize with the population you serve. If you decide to become a clinical instructor, your students will need your ears to listen to their concerns.

Compassion will give your nursing career longevity. I have a colleague and mentor who has been a nurse for over thirty years. She has a wealth of knowledge and energy. She keeps all of us on our toes! I've watched her care for her patients and I've listened to her stories. I particularly remember the stories she has shared about patients over the years, patients she loved who passed away.

I have often thought, *What keeps her going as a such a caring and energetic nurse for all these years?* Perhaps it's the genuine concern she shows for all of her patients. I think that her compassion gives her strength on tired days. It gives her words when she might not think she has any. I also think it helps her maintain energy when another career sounds tempting. Compassion has been with her for over thirty years as a nurse and it still shows brightly in the care of her patients.

Believe it or not, compassion can fix a shift that has gone wrong. I remember it like it was yesterday. I stood in the middle of my patient's room while the grandmother read me the riot act. She said some truly mean things to me. I cried, almost to the point of audible sobs. After she finished laying into me, I quietly left the room and spent the next half an hour composing myself so I could finish my shift.

As you progress in your nursing career, you will have times when you feel like you can't please your patients or their families no matter what you do. What do you do in those moments? Particularly in those moments when you're reduced to tears?

Well, I went back into the room and continued to care for the patient to best of my ability. I made sure to smile, show kindness, and listen to all the family's concerns. When the shift ended, the grandmother came to me with a hug and an apology!

Compassion can literally transform bad situations for you! Before my run-in with this family member, I took a task oriented approach with the patient's care. I didn't take the time I needed to listen to the family and show that I cared. But once I did, what began as a very sour shift turned around. I felt more confident in my ability to care for the patient.

It's very easy to think of "compassion" as a touchy-feely phrase that means you feel sorry for others' troubles. But I've discovered that it truly is an action word! To show compassion not only means to sympathize with patients and families, but also to work to ease their troubles. Think about how your actions will look to the patient in the bed, or to those by the bedside.

When you have a patient burning up with fever, you may feel compelled to do more than just get medicine. You'll want to try to a cool rag, cool liquids, and anything else you can think of to help make them comfortable. That's good—the little things we do make a difference. Practice the "own it" principle of compassionate nursing. It's a simple principle that means you will address a need for any patient, regardless of whether or not they are assigned to you. The scenario I have experienced has been something like this: I am running around with about five tasks to complete and ten thoughts in my mind. I'm headed to my patient's room when I'm stopped by a guest who asks me to get juice for the patient in another room. Since I'm busy, the first response that comes to mind is, "I'll let your nurse know". The problem with this response is that I might have just left someone with the impression that I am too busy to handle their small request.

The reality is that patients just want to be taken good care of, no matter how busy we are. What they remember most is someone cared enough to pause from being busy to address a need! So I will "own it" and grab the patient some juice. What a difference this can make in their perception of care!

I remember a family that particularly moved one of my colleagues. She went to the hospital shop and came back with a special gift for the patient. She gave the patient a gift they had always wanted, but never had—because the family couldn't afford it. When my colleague presented the gift, the entire family, including the patient, cried with gratitude and happiness. I thought, *What a difference a determination to help someone can make!* My colleague looked at me and said, "This is why we are here."

I will never forget the experience. You've chosen to be a nurse, so you are probably hardwired to show compassion. You will have patients who will tug at your heart strings; you may you feel compelled to go the extra mile to help them. Do it! That's exactly how showing compassion looks.

If you really want to grow into the best nurse you ever thought you could be, base decisions on your concern for the patients. I once read that a nurse has a duty to his or her patient above all others in the care setting. That's pretty powerful! Take it to heart, especially as a new nurse and watch how awesome your nursing care becomes!

2

ROUTINE ORDERS?!

What You Can Expect To Experience as a New Grad and What To Take From It

"There are no ordinary moments. There is always something going on."

– Peaceful Warrior

You will experience many things during your first six months to a year of nursing practice, things that will seem ordinary, but will certainly test your wits. I'm going to take some time to detail what those incidents might be and what you can take away from them.

Rudeness

I would love to tell you that you will never encounter rudeness as a new nurse, but I will shoot for the truth instead. Rudeness will be yours to deal with at some point. It may come from doctors, patients, or shockingly, from your colleagues. You'll encounter it when you least expect it—sometimes when you feel like you cannot handle it.

Some mornings I've come into my patient's room, bright-eyed, smiling, and confident that the day will go well, only to meet with a patient in the most sour mood, evident by the constant cursing. I've also called a doctor, thinking that he would surely appreciate me clarifying his orders, only to hang up the phone, thinking, *What was that attitude all about?* When I started my nursing career, I didn't think I'd have to deal with all sorts of crankiness. But, since then, I have learned a few things about the aftermath of rudeness.

You may never know the reason behind someone's short tone or cranky mood, but you will know how you respond best to it. You may be someone who cries when angry. Perhaps you're known for confronting situations head-on, if you catch my drift. However you normally deal with rudeness, be sure to keep a cool head. If you get that sudden urge to match the person's attitude with one of your own, resist! You may say something you will regret or get a reputation for being snippy.

Look at it this way: hospitals, or any area where medicine is practiced, can be stressful. People might not always act the way you think they should. Your job is to be prepared for it. Be determined to keep showing kindness when met with hostility or a short temper. You won't always feel like it, believe me, but you'll see your patience level increase and you'll be a better nurse for it!

Priorities...Priorities...

When you're in nursing school, giving medications is great! You spend time learning about the medication, talking about it with the nursing instructor and going to give it right when it is due. It may not always go that smoothly when you start nursing in the field. I once had a colleague ask me, "Have you ever looked up at the clock and realized you forgot to give a medication?" Another colleague and I quickly responded, "Sure. It happens!"

You will have shifts when you need to work a little harder at prioritizing to get things done on time. Will giving a medication late mean you should march immediately to your manager to submit your resignation? Of course not! But it could mean a number of other things.

First, if you're going through your shift imagining a red cape hanging from your scrubs, you've probably got a super-nurse complex to get over. Sometimes you won't be able to do it all! Teamwork is a wonderful thing; so be sure to use it. Ask for help when you need to. Your first year in nursing is a great time to learn this.

I once worked a shift when, the more I got done, the more new orders I had to complete. I didn't really ask for help because I thought, *I'll look I like can't handle myself* or *I'll be a burden to my teammates*. Well, the shift marched on. At five that evening, I still had not eaten lunch (the shift ended at seven), and in my mind I was screaming, *Help me!* Things would have been so much easier if I just asked a teammate for help.

It's dangerous to become so focused on caring for your patients that you don't reach out to others working with you. I'll give you a scenario I've seen many times.

You're caring for a patient whose condition has been getting worse for hours during your shift. Most of your time has been spent at this patient's bedside. You've been watching over this patient like a hawk, and you're feeling pretty good about your care. Your other patients are doing okay. Some of your other medications are now late in administration, but that's okay. You're still on top of things, right?

Suddenly, the patient you are focused on starts to get worse. Doctors appear at the bedside, asking you to give several medications, do frequent reassessments, and then immediately transfer the patient to another unit for increased monitoring. This may not sound that bad, but I can guarantee that, if this happens to you as a new nurse, you're going to want some help at the bedside.

Take a closer look at this scenario. Suppose you had asked your fellow nurses to give any medications due for your other patients? Suppose the charge nurse or team leader had known how busy you were with the sicker patient? His or help could have been invaluable to you when it was time to follow the doctor's orders and transport the patient to the other unit.

Help can make the difference. Help can also save your patient. I had an episode with a patient that I will never forget. I had just got the patient back from the recovery unit and I was completing an assessment when the patient threw up a large amount of bright red blood. The patient's blood pressure dropped, so I knew it was time to call for help. Before I could blink, I, my teammate, and a nursing leader working on the unit had given the patient fluid boluses several times, started another IV, had blood prepared, and were rushing the patient back to the operating room! All of this happened with the entire physician team at the bedside.

I cannot begin to imagine what might have happened if I had not had the extra pairs of hands helping me. I will be forever grateful to my fellow nurse, who put off taking her lunch break to help me! I was not a super-nurse that day. I was a nurse who was gravely concerned for her patient, and called for help because I knew I could not handle it alone.

You may not be quite sure what to do first when you have several tasks. That is okay in your first year because you are learning. No one expects you to come in on roller skates. Again, be sure to ask for advice and help if you're unsure about task management. You'll see that the old saying is true: there is safety in numbers.

Night Shifts, Holidays and Weekends

Adjusting to a nurse's schedule as a new graduate can be so tough. The idea of walking and thinking at three in the morning still makes me nervous. How I hated working the night shift! I always felt like I had been hit by a large truck the next morning. No amount of caffeine helped at all; I had to drive home with the windows down to stay reasonably alert. Thankfully, after a year or two, I was able to move to working dayshift only.

I also remember seeing a holiday track as a new graduate. Our holiday track shows what holidays we're assigned to work for the year. When I first noticed that I would be working Thanksgiving and Christmas, I wanted to cry! I had never missed spending those holidays with my family before. Thankfully, my teammates and the hospital-wide activities made working holidays better. There's usually lots of laughter on the holidays.

You may very well be asked to work on holidays you love celebrating with family and friends. You may have to adjust to working nightshifts and weekend shifts that seem to drain your social life. In all honesty, it sucks sometimes. But there's good news! There are some things to keep in mind when your schedule is not quite the way you want it.

* Pay your dues. There may be some schedule woes you have to deal with when you're new. It's all a part of paying dues. Once you gain some seniority, you may be able to have more input in your schedule. But in the meantime, take comfort in knowing that it is a temporary situation.

* Potlucks, residents, and late night chats can make a nightshift not only bearable, but fun! Find out what makes those undesirable shifts work and make the most of it. I remember when an anonymous family would donate insanely large amounts of food to hospital staff, patients, and families on Thanksgiving. It was great for those of us working to be able to share in the festivities. Maybe you and your teammates can bring food and gifts on holidays. Secret Santas and Halloween costume contests make units cheerful places on holidays. If it will help to cheer you up, participate!

*Learn the art of negotiation! There will probably be a colleague who needs to tweak their schedule and wouldn't mind swapping a shift with you. To get a successful swap, keep some things in mind. Be sure to state why you need a swap. While one colleague may swap with you out of sheer kindness, another may be wondering why they should re-arrange their routine to help you. Leave no room for guessing. Also, be confident. Try to go to as many people directly as you can. I've tried to arrange swaps by sending out mass emails to staff, but that method is not direct enough to get success. So be prepared to have face-to-face conversation with your colleagues to get those shift swaps. Last, be sure to let your colleagues know that you will return the favor. It might given them extra incentive to swap with you

No Lunch?!?

I want to say briefly that I don't mean to scare anyone or exaggerate about how busy nursing shifts can be. I just want to be sure that I present all the possibilities of what could happen when things get busy; unfortunately, going the shift without lunch can happen! If you're not careful, you can keep going and going, all the while thinking, *I'll take a break as soon as I....* But as the shift goes on and your tasks keep coming, that break time never comes. You might also experience a partial lunch, that is, a lunch break where you spend your time thinking and talking about patient care, so your brain never gets downtime.

So, what can you do to prevent accidental fasting on your shifts? Here's a few tips! The first is fairly basic. Bring snacks. Your shifts can be physically, mentally, and emotionally demanding. Snacks will keep you going on those shifts when you may not get to break for lunch at an ideal time. Your unit may have a "snack fund" that you all contribute to.

Next, plan ahead. As you learn how to prioritize your tasks, you'll find planning your lunch breaks useful. Share your planned lunch break with your charge nurse or team leader. That way, you make sure someone is available to help you stay on task and take your break. You should also let someone know when you are going on break, so that your patients are covered.

If at all possible, take your break off your unit. As wonderful as break rooms can be, they don't always give you that quiet time you need to recharge for the rest of your shift. When it was possible, I would love to just go, sit, and take deep breaths in the hospital's garden. I really felt ready to complete my shift when the break ended. Even if your care setting does not have a garden, do your best to take your breaks in areas you find calming. Trust me, you'll notice the difference when you return to the floor.

Finally, try not to talk about patient care during your break. It's called a break for a reason! Your mind needs a chance to pause for a few minutes. Don't use your break time to rant and rave about the craziness of the shift. Will this be hard? Absolutely, but do your best.

Remember, your break time is for you. Be sure to use it so it benefits you.

Boundaries

Nursing is such a special profession. You meet and befriend the most interesting people, and some of them will be forever grateful for the care you give them. You will treasure these experiences and the bonds you form while caring for them. Throughout my nursing career, I've come to care a great deal for some of my patients and families. It has not always been easy to tell if I have crossed a professional boundary line. I've found myself in positions where I just wanted to fix it, fix everything that was wrong. I wanted to lecture parents who could care for their chronically ill children better. I wanted to lash out at patients who weren't taking care of themselves at home. In your nursing career, you will face this same question: ***Where is the professional boundary line and have I crossed it?***

Nurse Katy, for example, cares for senior patients in a nursing home. One of her particular patients, Mr. Wilson, reminds Katy of her own father. Katy spends extra time with Mr. Wilson after her shift ends, she eats her meals with him, and sometimes she visits him on holidays. When Mr. Wilson passes, Katy grieves, but finds it very difficult to accept Mr. Wilson's death. When Katy starts to have trouble forming relationships with new patients, her colleagues and friends recommend counseling for her.

What do you think of Katy's nursing situation? Scenarios like this happen more often than you may expect. Hospitals usually have guidelines on things like accepting gifts from patients, ethical behavior, and so forth. It speaks volumes about our profession that nurses touch others' lives so deeply. But remember, you will, like Katy, involve your heart when caring for your patients. Professional boundaries are often clear, but sometimes they're a fine line, especially when you've formed a bond with a patient. You may cross that fine line sometime. Here are a few helpful tips to help you stay within the lines of professionalism and maintain healthy relationships with your patients.

Keep your memories in a special place. When the boundaries blur, we run into danger by not appreciating our relationships with our patients, not grieving properly when patients pass, and not allowing our emotions to heal.

I have colleagues who have been pediatric nurses for a very long time. They've absolutely fallen in love with the children they've cared for, and some of those children have passed away. I've heard other nurses describing how they store the memories of these special children in keepsake boxes or scrapbooks. What a great way to keep the memories! They've kept cards, pictures, drawings, things to remind them of the special moments they had with their patients. Storing your memories will help you remember, in a healthy way, the lives you have impacted, and those who've impacted yours. Will it sometimes be heartbreaking to care for your patients?

Yes, but you can remember those relationships in a good way, with fondness.

Don't judge. It's in your nature as a nurse to want to help and fix things. Conviction, zeal, and knowledge are the traits that make you a remarkable gift to your patients and families. You will have to know when and how to approach them. You must remain professional, about confrontational issues in particular. I've met parents who have asthmatic children, yet smoke inside of the house. As a nurse who wants what's best for her patient, suppose I march into my patient's room and give the parents a stern lecture about the hazards of smoking. Am I doing what's necessary as a healthcare professional or am I being judgmental without examining all the details? Have the parents been lectured before? Have they tried to quit before? What obstacles do they face?

For these types of situations, I've used the **think and listen** method. It works! Here's what you do:

• **Think!** Is it in the patient's best interest to be confronted about this issue at this time? Be sure to collect all the details about the situation. Is there some history or special circumstances to be aware of? Consider carefully all points of view on the subject. Rationality is a great tool!

• **Listen!** While your patient or a family member explains the situation, actively listen. This means that you probably don't want to have any preconceived notions about what they're going to say. Who knows? While you're listening, you might hear some new details on the situation that you didn't consider, which may change your entire approach. In the example of the parents who smoke, suppose there was a recent stressor in their lives such as job loss or family member's death that prompted the smoking? You probably won't learn those things unless you listen attentively. Also, you'll discover that they may not need a lecture at that moment, just someone to listen and care.

• *Know your role!* You may care for patients who have heard everything there is to hear about their health. They've heard all the lectures, warnings, and advice, yet still fail to care for themselves properly. Sometimes, your smile or comforting hand can be just as supportive as all of the healthcare advice in the world! Your role at that point may be just to be supportive. You can listen to your patients' concerns and support them in how they choose to take to care of themselves. Dealing with a chronic illness on a daily basis while trying to maintain some normalcy has to be very difficult. Your role can simply be to show them that you are listening to them and that you care.

The Beautiful Goodbyes

As a nurse, you will experience some things that no amount of schooling can fully prepare you for. The death of a patient is one of those things. You may care for patients who are chronically ill, whose deaths don't come so suddenly. Some patients you may lose unexpectedly. However and whenever it happens, I hope to somehow prepare you a little for what you may experience. I can shed some light on what I call "beautiful goodbyes", when you and your team grieve together and console each other when patients die.

Be willing to share with others. Grief and loss bring people together. You'll witness the support of fellow staff members, friends, and sometimes family members of the patients you've lost. I remember when my colleagues and I said goodbye to a patient we had loved and taken care of for years. I received a phone call from one of my co-workers letting me know that the patient would pass soon. I drove up to the hospital, meeting several of my teammates in the room. We all stood by the bedside, where we took turns saying our goodbyes. We spent time consoling each other and recalling our favorite memories of the patient. It was such a tough day and I was never quite sure I could again handle losing another patient to a terrible disease. I remember my teammates and I leaning on each other in such a way that made the situation easier to deal with.

Another time, my teammates and I received a phone call from the intensive care unit. One of our frequent long-term patients had just died. My teammates and I went to the ICU room to comfort the family and say our goodbyes. I'll never forget how peaceful the patient looked or how grateful the family was that we came down to be with them. Despite our shared sadness, both of these were wonderful times of closeness and healing for those of us on the staff. As painful as goodbyes will be for you, count yourself fortunate that you'll have colleagues, friends and family to help you heal. That kind of bond helps make those goodbyes all the more beautiful.

Losing your patients may make you wonder if you can handle forming strong bonds with other patients. I know nurses who have cared for terminally ill patients for a great number of years. What they've frequently shared with me is the importance of knowing your personal limits. So I'll share their advice with you: know how much you, personally, can handle. If the grief begins to affect your work, mood, or personal life, it could indicate that you have reached your limit. Reaching your limit doesn't mean that you are not able to care for patients any longer, but it could mean that you need help with processing your grief. Learn to recognize if and how grief is affecting you at work. You could also explore other avenues of nursing for a short period of time. No matter what, you have to maintain your emotional health to be the best nurse you can be.

3

SCRUBS!

Recognize Your Teammates and Learn to Make the Most of Teamwork

"A successful team beats with one heart"

-Unknown

Simply put, teamwork is more valuable than all of the technical skills you learn in nursing school put together. Lack of it can make for a difficult shift, but the right amount of it can make your shift sail smoothly! As you get going into your nursing practice, here are some tips on teamwork and how it will benefit you on the job.

Speak up! If you're drowning in work, yet no one knows, how will you survive? The answer is that you may not for long. Continued stress and hectic environments can wreak havoc on your morale. You also don't want to allow your patients' care to be affected by your overload. So for your sake and your patients' sake, be upfront about needing help.

Recognize who's in your corner! It's true what they say: no man is an island. To care adequately for a patient, it takes a team of doctors, nurses, care techs, social workers, case managers, etc., all giving their best efforts on the patient's behalf. Be sure to value the input you'll get from your care team members. Don't be shy. Give your input as well! It may make all the difference in your patient's outcomes.

Reach out to your teammates! When you're just trying to get through your shift, it can be so easy to hide yourself in a corner to chart, write things down, or even think. If you find that you've been in your corner a while, look up and check on your teammates. Make sure that no one needs your help. If you take the time to help others, you will notice your teammates returning the favor. You will also gain a reputation as a team player and garner much more respect from colleagues.

Set clear expectations for help.. You'll have great patient care technicians/associates to help you care for patients. Set clear expectations to make your partnership as effective as possible. You'll save time, energy and frustration if you are specific about the help you need. I'll call this tip the art of delegation. Be specific about what you need, as well as how and when you need it. Try not to leave any guesswork when you delegate tasks and make sure the tasks are appropriate for delegation. Of course, this is a simplified mention of delegation and you'll learn far more about the subject in your care setting.

Who's On Your Team?

As you get more accustomed to caring for your patients, begin to pay more and more attention to the team of people who help you and just how important your relationship with them is. So here's a brief list of the people who will come to be very important in the effective care of your patient. You might be surprised at the role they will play in helping you have a good shift!

The Communication Center

First up, let's look at the hub of your unit's communication—the unit secretary. If you don't believe the secretary is central to good patient care, just wait until you work a shift without one! Having to answer calls, filter communication, and sort documents in between giving medications, making beds, and performing all your other tasks will give you a whole new appreciation of the unit secretary by your shift's end!

Your unit secretary helps with everything from making sure your patients' needs are addressed in a timely fashion to determining which calls are most important. You will need to know how to make the most out of your work relationship with the secretary.

For starters, let the secretary know where you're going. When you step away from the nurses' station, letting the secretary know where you are headed and how long you'll be gone ensures that others will know that you're off the floor. Let's say a doctor comes up looking for you, but none of the other team members know where you've gone. If you've checked in with the secretary, he or she can speak up and save you from being overhead paged and hunted down for a good ten minutes.

Also—this may seem simple—but be sure to let your secretary know when you've paged someone! I can't tell you the number of missed phone calls I've seen, simply because the nurse stepped away from the nurses' station without letting the secretary know to expect a page return. The most important thing you can do for the unit secretary is keep them updated. If they are in the loop, it improves communication throughout the entire unit.

The Lung Specialist

The next team member can probably show you all kinds of ways to induce coughing and you will definitely want to have them on your side during the winter season! Meet the respiratory therapist. I've cared for patients with cystic fibrosis and asthma, so needless to say, I know the vast importance of a respiratory care professional on the care team. They are knowledgeable and greatly committed to doing what's best for the patients. They also serve as wonderful advocates for the patient's needs. So, the best advice I can give you is this: listen to your respiratory care professional! When you note that your patient is in respiratory distress, be sure to call the RCP, even if it is just to gain some of their input on how to intervene for the patient. Two heads are always better than one, and they will more than likely appreciate your keeping them posted on what is going on. Also, help them advocate for the patient. When the RCP brings a patient's need to your attention, discuss it with the physician if the RCP doesn't have the time. This way, you're making patient advocacy a team effort, which is always a plus! Here are a few other times to be sure to call your respiratory therapist

• Your patient's not breathing right! It sounds like common sense, right? Well, you might be surprised. When you're in those situations where your patient has trouble breathing, your adrenaline kicks in and you intervene. Calling the RCP for backup may be the last thing on your mind. So this is just a little reminder to call the cavalry when the need arises.

• If the doctor orders new respiratory medications for your patient that you may not be too familiar with, that would be a good time to talk about the medication with the therapist. You will more than likely learn something new that will enhance your nursing practice.

The Doctor

Truth be told, the days of house calls have passed. Doctors practicing in hospitals have to be time- and cost-effective when caring for patients, all the while maintaining a sufficient knowledge base, safe patient care, and good leadership skills. Their responsibilities are tremendous!

Thankfully, you as the nurse are there to support them as a member of the care team. Your relationship to the doctor is a unique one. I like to think of it like this: if the care team is a body, then the physician is the head and you as the nurse represent the hands, legs, and heart. You both will have to function together perfectly in your roles to properly care for your patient.

Neither the heart nor the brain, the legs nor the arms can operate alone. One of best things you can do for your patient is to work with the doctor, not view him or her as an adversary. There will be times when you have a different idea about how care for the patient, but be sure to present your thoughts to the physician in a respectful manner. Try not to act as if you know better or be defensive. Doing that will put your relationship with the doctor in danger of becoming unproductive, which probably won't lead to the best outcome for your patient.

I once had a confrontation with a doctor that I regret to this very day. I paged the physician because I was concerned for my patient who had persistent breathing problems. When I spoke with the doctor, her clipped tone and short answers made it seem as if receiving the page had annoyed her. Her tone shocked me, so I decided to let her know in the middle of phone call how it was rude, unnecessary, unappreciated, etc. Needless to say, our conversation did not start well when she reached the floor. I am grateful it ended in mutual apologies and a recovering of our relationship, but, looking back, I did something that I will not make the mistake of doing again. I won't go on the defensive.

I also forgot to keep the patient first. The encounter I had with the doctor flooded my thoughts, pushing out what was going on with my patient. If I had to page the doctor for anything else after I got defensive, it would have been uncomfortable talking to her.

The bottom line is that strife between you and the doctor will, more likely than not, put good patient care in jeopardy. So try to remain calm and put your patient's care at the front of your mind.

The Colleague

You'll laugh, cry, and vent together. There'll be birthdays, weddings, holiday parties, promotions, baby showers, and more discussions about diets and dating than you ever thought possible! Your fellow nurses and co-workers are an important part of your team for a very special reason: they get it. Try explaining the craziness of your shift to your family members and then see what I mean. Sure, they empathize with your exhaustion, but they don't fully get what you mean when you explain taking a fifteen minute lunch break, getting fussed at by a doctor, losing two IVs, spilling your blood after you spiked the bag, and the list goes on and on.

Your colleagues are also there to support you. You will need their strength on tough days and vice versa. My teammates and I have learned to watch for each other's "stress cues." As you work more with your colleagues, some who become your best friends, you'll be able to tell when they're under a high level of stress.

You probably think that will be easy, huh? Well, not always. We all react differently under stress. We may have a different tone of voice or different body language. We may be irritable, emotional, or flat. The point is that your teammates will learn your signs and you will learn theirs. It's a great asset!

I'll never forget a shift when I had a patient throwing up blood with dropping blood pressures. I had given some fluid and the doctors were on the way up to assess the patient. My teammate saw me in the hallway and asked if I was ready to go on our lunch break like we had planned earlier. Well, she looked at my face and my patient's blood pressure on the monitor. Her next statement to me was, "What can I do to help you?"

Before I knew it, she was on her way to pick up blood for my patient while I stayed at the bedside with the doctors getting ready to rush the patient to the operating room. What stuck out in my mind is that I did not have to say, "Help me". I had worked with my friend for years and she could tell by the look on my face that I needed help! As you begin your nursing practice, value the role you play in helping your colleagues. Your teamwork will make the difference in how a difficult shift is handled.

The Patient

If there is any one person essential to your care team—and even to your growth in your first year of nursing—it's the person I'm about to mention. I would even dare to say that, if you don't form a good relationship with this person, your practice and growth as a nurse will be hindered. That person is none other than your patient.

If you're going to have any impact or grow successfully as a bedside clinician, you have to seek a relationship with your patient. Several of my patients have chronic illnesses that require them to stay in the hospital for extended periods of time. So much of care for these patients centers on the bonds formed with them. I've seen firsthand how a nurse has improved care for a patient because they had a good relationship. One of our frequent patients, who was well-known and a favorite of one of my colleagues, came in for a two-week stay. We were reviewing the patient's medication orders and my colleague noticed that one of the patient's home medications had been ordered incorrectly. The problem was quickly corrected, but just think of how much their nurse-patient relationship improved the patient's care! Your technical skills will improve as you go on, but your listening and advocacy skills will only strengthen as you strengthen your relationships with your patients.

I once had a nursing professor tell me that she prefers for her nursing students to spend their downtime talking to the patient and family. It shows your patient that you have an active interest in what's going on with them. It also sharpens your ability to listen and form relationships with patients, one of the key skills you can build as a new nurse. I'll never forget that lesson. I hope you take it with you as well.

4

THE TIP JAR

Finish Your First Year of Practice Strong

"The biggest room in the world is the room for improvement"

- Author Unknown

In addition to compassion, another large part of heart nursing is confidence. Resist the urge to be hard on yourself! As a nurse, you're in a constant state of learning and growth. That's wonderful news for your patients. Growth for you means better care for them. Keep that in the front of your minds during orientation, classes and competency training. Especially keep it in mind when things go wrong. Confidence is key to your growth as a new nurse. The truth is, it often shows to the patient when you are new, especially when there is a new skill to learn.

Once when I was learning to start IV's, I had some difficulty finding a patient's vein with the IV catheter. The patient was in tears and the doctor was at the bedside, waiting on successful IV placement. Suddenly a family member told the patient, "It's okay, we have to just deal with new people". I was mortified. To make matters worse, another nurse with more IV experience comes into the room, and I could literally hear the sighs of relief from the patient, family and the doctor! I left the room overwhelmed with defeat, certain that I never wanted to try an IV again. I then remembered what a mentor once told me. "If you want to be good at IV's, keep sticking". Her advice encouraged me to be confident in my abilities and persistent in mastering new skills.

I share the same advice with you. Keep at the skill. You may do it differently from other nurses, and that is okay. The point is that you will learn. No matter how long it takes you to master the nursing skill, remember that you are intelligent and capable.

It Could Happen To You

Here are some mishaps that I've seen happen during steady and busy shifts. I've even experienced a few of these myself. They make no sense, are often unexplainable and occasionally make for longer shifts. You might feel less intelligent or frazzled when you experience one, but relax. Many of us have felt that way! Remember that even the best nurse is not immune to mishaps. Mishaps are growing opportunities! They suck, but good can come out of them. What's important is that you keep learning.

1. You've been told several times to be careful when spiking blood bags. You've pre-medicated the patient, picked up the blood from blood bank and gotten another nurse to witness the unit. What happens next? You spike a hole right through the bag.

2. You go to hang an IV medication. You verify your pump settings and press start on the pump. You head to the nurses' station, feeling so on top of things. You go back to flush your medication and notice a puddle on the floor. Much to your surprise, you forgot to actually connect the tubing to the patient's IV.

3. You're in the middle of change of shift report, preparing to review your assessment with the oncoming nurse. As you skim the chart, you notice that you didn't chart your assessment or intake and output for the shift.

4. Your patient needs a central line dressing change and lab draws. You change the dressing and flush the line with heparin, afterwards realizing you forgot to draw the labs.

5. You get morning vital signs on your patient, but don't write them down because you plan to record them from the monitor a little later. "Later" arrives and you go to record the vital signs, only to discover the monitor has been turned off and all previous data lost.

6. You tell your charge nurse that you are going on your lunch break. You report that your patients will not need anything while you are gone. As your

food is warming, you get notified that one of your patients is febrile, another on the way back from the OR and a there's a doctor who would like to clarify some orders with you.

7. The doctor informs the patient that they are being discharged during your shift. When you go into the patient's room with discharge paperwork to be signed, you discover the patient has left.

8. Your patient is very nauseous, so you rush to get an emesis bin. Unfortunately, you're not quick enough and your good scrub pants are ruined.

9. A new patient arrives. You didn't know they are assigned to you and you haven't even sat to chart on your other patients.

10. You go into the patient's room to start an IV. You're met with the question, "Are you any good at this"?

There are many more that deserve honorable mention, some of which you'll experience. Just remember that in the pace of your shifts, things will happen. Here's how best to deal with them: Stay confident in your skills as a nurse, keep a good attitude, learn to laugh at yourself and keep your cool!

Myths & Legends

If you ask around, perceptions of nurses are typically pretty positive. There are occasionally some scary images of ladies in white with huge needles, but overall, nurses are highly regarded. When you picture a nurse you admire, traits like kind, compassionate, patient and organized probably come to mind. I've always admired the stories of Florence Nightingale. Her compassion, intelligence and foresight made nursing seem like a career for heroes! Picturing yourself as a nurse of this caliber is awesome. It means that you indeed will be. But not every nurse feels like a hero all the time. You may run into some letdowns and unmet expectations if no one dispels the myths of nurse legend for you. Here are a few I would like to highlight.

Myth #1: **You're a beacon of kindness and compassion who is slow to get angry and quick to be patient.** I laughed while writing this! Allow me to share this reality with you: There will be times when you're cranky and impatient. You will get tired of hearing your name called. You won't feel up to smiling and it will be hard for you not to judge the non-compliant patient who's back in the hospital after being discharged a few weeks earlier. Sometimes, you will want to just do the bare minimum of nursing and go home. Does this mean you're a bad nurse? Of course not. You are still a beacon, just a human one.

Myth # 2: **You never resent or feel guilty for having to leave your family to take care of others.** This is a tough one! I've heard several nurses comment on how hard it is sometimes to leave their loved ones, especially if they're sick, to care for patients. In all honesty, you might question how fair it is to your family and your patients.

How great of care can you give if you're worried about your family? Oh, and new mommies, prepare yourselves for possible tears the first time you leave your baby to report back to work. But don't be alarmed by all of this. I've seen many deal with these kind of tough choices and still be rockstar nurses to patients. It all works out! The wisest thing to do is always know what's best for you and your family. Be able to recognize if resentment is affecting your practice.

Myth #3: **You are flexible and open to change.** A big part of gaining confidence as a nurse is building a routine and mastering it. You learn to feel good about performing a skill because you do it a certain way over and over again. It eventually becomes second nature. So what happens next? Research shows there's a better way to do the skill, hospital policy changes and you're basically back to learning a new routine. (insert scream here). Your next statement might go something like this, "The hospital policy is changing?! I just learned how to do this!" No worries. You'll more than likely find a colleague who shares your pain! What helps build flexibility is if you keep at the forefront of your mind the reason for the change: better patient care. Change is inevitable, especially when excellence is the goal.

Myth #4: **You are super organized and together**. I've had shifts where I looked back and wondered how I got it all done. All meds were given, procedures done and new orders completed. I think sometimes, I really need to apply some of this efficiency to house cleaning! Dishes are in the sink, the fridge is empty and my car needs maintenance. On top of that, my motivation level to handle those things sometimes is slim to none, especially after working a crazy shift. I'm sure I'm not alone. You won't be either. You would be surprised at how many of us nurses are so gifted at taking care of others when our own lives are a mess! If you find yourself in this situation, remember to cut yourself a little slack. It's okay to not have everything neat and in its place in your life sometimes.

21 Tips for Your Learning and Growing

These tips have helped me so much, beyond novice level nursing and even into other areas of my life. Read them, laugh at them and most importantly, practice them!

1. Be confident! Being new can be scary, but you can handle it.

2. Listen attentively, especially to your patient. Carve out time in your shift to talk with their family. You're more likely to take better care of them.

3. Who on your unit has been there the longest? Be sure to get to know that person if you can. They will have a wealth of knowledge and wisdom for you to learn.

4. Count no skill as useless. Learn to do as much as you can. You'll be an invaluable asset to your patients, team, and unit.

5. If you begin to hear the infusion pump alarms from work at home, don't worry! It happens to a lot of us.

6. It's okay to rehearse what you're going to say before you call the doctor. No one should judge you.

7. Doing a procedure at the bedside? Grab everything you need in one trip. I can't tell you how much extra work you can create for yourself by having to go and get materials you forgot to bring to the bedside the first time.

8. Whatever you do, don't get a reputation as a complainer! It's a hard reputation to shake. If something frustrates you, find the appropriate channel to share your concerns.

9. Do you have an idea for something you'd like to see done differently? Share it! The greatest changes have come from someone passionate enough to act on an idea!

10. Never utter the words "It's a quiet shift right now." Once you've said that, it may not be quiet for long!

11. Write it all down. Until you get the hang of managing tasks and thoughts, jot down as much as you can. When your shift is over and the adrenaline comes down, your mind may not have held on to as much information as you would like

12. Get, have, and keep a life! Loving and caring for your patients can be consuming. So can hospital affairs. Preserve your sanity and be sure to have a good work-life balance.

13. You won't know it all. I repeat, you won't know it all. But a willingness to learn will attract those who want to teach you. You'll be better for it.

14. Don't dwell too long on your mistakes. They happen, and it's tough when they affect the patient. Ask yourself the important questions after the mistake is made (i.e., What did I learn from this? How can I improve things so this mistake doesn't happen again?) and then move on.

15. Value other care team members' roles. Collaborate with them about your patient's care as often as you can.

16. Find joy in simple things. It will help to keep your heart hopeful! A nurse who remains hopeful

17. Have a good wristwatch and a good pair of shoes!

18. Have a place to vent. You need somewhere you can go to let off steam and clear your head. If you feel tears coming on, go there and, if necessary, let a colleague know where you're going.

19. Do you know what your patient likes to called? Learn this! It's key to starting a good relationship with them.

20. Help out! You'll be surprised how much help will come to you when needed simply because you took time to help others.

21. Cherish every learning opportunity. Your first year of practice will fly by! Learn, laugh and grow as much as you can.

Change of Shift

So, you're on a wonderful journey. You'll see, do, and learn things that will shape the rest of your nursing career. Whether you are a nursing student or a novice, take full advantage of the place you are in! Ultimately, you are in control of the kind of nurse you will become. Soak it all in. Observe. Grow. Learn! Don't shrink back from any opportunity to better your skills. The landscape of nursing is changing and, the more you can do, the more valuable you are.

I will leave you with one last story. I was in my first year of practice and had just completed orientation. One of my patients was very sick and had a lot of orders like frequent labs, fluid titrations, increased monitoring, etc. You get the picture. I completed all of the doctor's orders and felt like I had done a good job after my shift was done. But while giving report to the next nurse, she discovered that I had given the wrong IV fluids to the patient. As sick as the patient was, this was a serious error. My heart dropped. I could have caused my patient harm.

On my next shift, my nurse manager asked me into her office to talk about the error. I expected her words to be something like this, "Please place your ID badge and stethoscope on my desk and kindly find the nearest exit". What she actually said has always stuck with me. *"Let's look back over the doctor's orders to see where you might have misunderstood something".* I was floored! I had just made a huge error (hence the meeting with the manager) and she actually took an opportunity to coach me. I was never made to feel small or like I wouldn't get the hang of things. The experience has always stuck with me. There are two things I learned from it that I want to leave with you.

First, the way my manager encouraged me actually made me want to perform at my best level! That taught me the power of encouragement. *Heart Nursing* is my way of encouraging you as a new nurse, especially in moments when you may not be sure that you chose the right career. Encouragement has a way of making you excel, even when you don't consider it possible. All that to say, you can do it!

Second, I learned what to say if a new graduate asked me what to expect as a new nurse. Expect laughter, tears, stress, anger, joy and a lot of other emotions, sometimes in the same shift! Expect to make mistakes, but let the mistakes build your character. Don't beat yourself up. If you really want to bounce back after a mistake, be a source of encouragement for the next nurse. It never hurts to pay it forward.

The essence of heart nursing is compassion. Your heart, hands, and mind are your most valuable tools. (Okay, so your feet are, too). But no matter what skills you harness, your ability to smile, think, and help is precious! Lean on those abilities the most, nurse from your heart and watch how others truly come to value you as a professional. What is even more rewarding is how you will value yourself as a professional nurse.

You could've chosen another profession, but you've chosen nursing, and what a choice you've made! You are a gift to your patients. Keep this in mind, and your first year of practice will be the start of a tremendous nursing career.

About the Author

AMANDA V. WEST is a registered pediatric nurse and motivational speaker to new and potential nurses. For more information about Amanda's speaking topics, upcoming books and blogs, visit her website:

www.amandavwest.com

Feel free to contact Amanda. She would love to get your feedback and answer any questions you may have about the profession of nursing.

amanda@amandavwest.com